Zoltan Rona MD MSc

Fighting Fibromyalgia

Natural help to reverse chronic pain

alive books

Vancouver
Canada

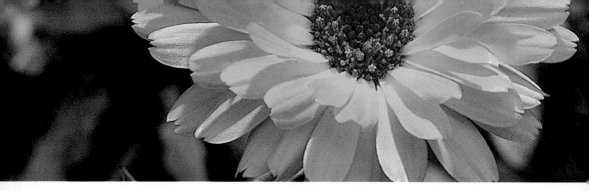

C o n t e n t s

All About Fibromyalgia

Note: Conversions in this book (from imperial to metric) are not exact. They have been rounded to the nearest measurement for convenience. Exact measurements are given in imperial. The recipes in this book are by no means to be taken as therapeutic. They simply promote the philosophy of both the author and *alive* books in relation to whole foods, health and nutrition, while incorporating the practical advice given by the author in the first section of the book.

Healthy Recipes

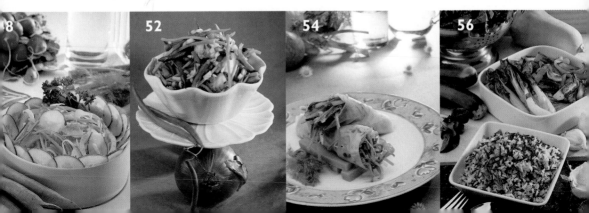

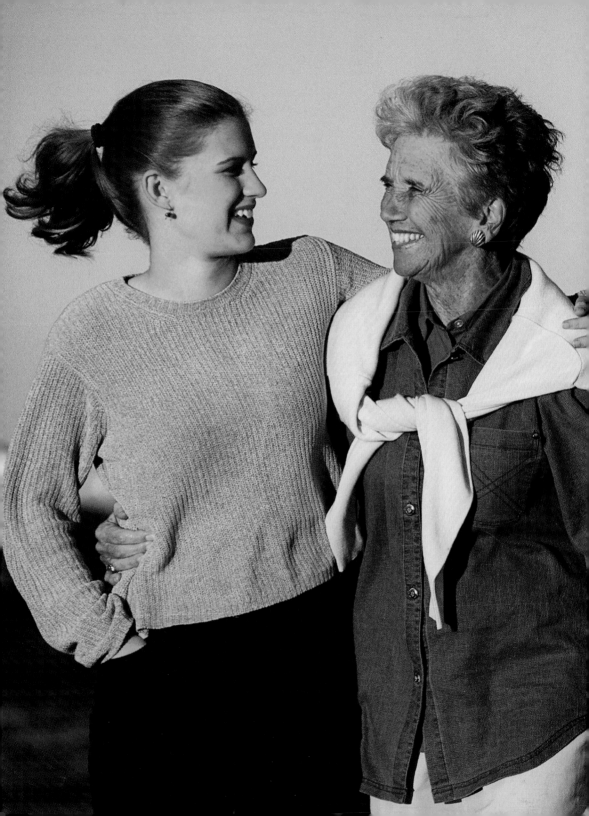

All About Fibromyalgia

To this day, many doctors still believe that Fibromyalgia is "all in your head." It isn't.

It's *Not* All in Your Head . . . .

Fibromyalgia is reversible.

It is estimated that between three and six million people in Canada and the United States suffer from Fibromyalgia. Of these people, about 80 percent are women between the ages of twenty and fifty. This chronic illness accounts for more than 5 percent of a doctor's practice and, for the most part, leaves the medical profession perplexed.

When I started in general practice in 1978, Fibromyalgia was a rare condition, perhaps worthy of a footnote in large medical texts but of little or no concern to most medical practitioners. In the mid-1980s, however, this changed dramatically. No one is completely sure what happened, but suddenly doctors began seeing an ever-growing number of people with multiple, non-specific complaints. These included chronic fatigue, sleep disturbances, generalized muscle and joint pains, intermittent flu-like illnesses, depression, anxiety, general malaise and cognitive impairment. With all these signs and symptoms occurring in the same individual at roughly the same time, doctors were baffled about both the diagnosis and how to treat the problem.

Initially, medical experts, who could find no evidence of bacterial, viral or other infection, theorized that this was a psychiatric illness, a form of depression. To this day, many doctors still believe that fibromyalgia is "all in your head." Aside from the psychiatric theory, speculation about the cause of the disorder has included Epstein-Barr virus infection (now disproven), a viral infection caused by type A influenza (possibly), hepatitis B vaccine reaction (unproven), chemical toxicity (controversial) and autoimmune disorder (most likely). The fact still remains that the disease is hard to diagnose, nearly impossible to distinguish from chronic fatigue syndrome and just as difficult to treat effectively. There is no blood test, x-ray or other accepted test that unequivocally diagnoses the condition.

The good news is that scientists are making advances in both diagnosis and treatment, mostly in the field of natural (complementary or integrative) medicine. As you are about to read in this book, Fibromyalgia is reversible if one follows a step-by-step approach using diet changes and other nutritional or biochemical balancing techniques. Regardless of what you have been told by the more pessimistic members of the medical profession, you can now take advantage of some of the latest

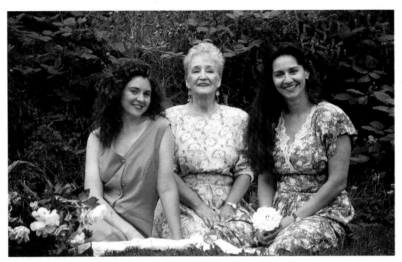

advancements and return to a normal or optimal state of health without taking dangerous drugs. Conventional medicine offers no cure for Fibromyalgia, however, many natural strategies and treatments do. All it takes in most cases is for people to become informed and take the initiative. And with this book you have a place to start doing just that.

Fibromyalgia is a condition that affects different generations.

Do You Hurt All Over? . . . .

Fibromyalgia is a syndrome, meaning that it involves the presence of many different signs and symptoms. People who suffer from Fibromyalgia Syndrome (FMS) do not share the same signs and symptoms equally but most complain that they "hurt all over." And nearly 100 percent of FMS victims report that they had some type of life event or life stressor just prior to the onset of the chronic pain.

Chronic pain disorder was first described in the medical literature in 1824. It was not until the 1980s, however, that it started to become more prominent as a diagnosis. Still, patients who consult natural health care practitioners continue to report that conventional medical doctors tell them it's all in their heads and they will just have to learn to live with it. And medical doctors, at least those in Canada, continue to refer FMS patients to psychiatrists regardless of the fact that FMS is not a psychiatric condition.

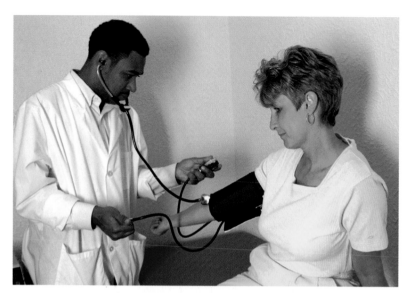

Fibromyalgia sufferers usually endure a battery of tests that do not explain their pain.

The Diagnostic Treadmill . . . .

Medical doctors attempt to look for the cause of pain before treating the patient. Unfortunately, with chronic pain disorders like FMS the usual course of action is to order various standard lab tests and then, when nothing is found on these tests to explain the pain, the patient is referred to a specialist of one kind or another. Most general practitioners will initially refer a chronic pain patient to a specialist in internal medicine whom then does further tests that show nothing abnormal. Then the internist, having nothing but drugs to offer to suppress pain, refers the patient to a psychiatrist or to a pain clinic. Once the patient has been shunted to these end-stage specialists, no one makes any further attempts to look for the cause of the pain.

Most FMS patients are not hypochondriacs or whiners but are suffering from demonstrable physical and mental dysfunction associated with disturbed sleep patterns and immune system abnormalities. The usual complaints of those suffering from FMS are aching and stiffness with multiple points of tenderness in numerous muscle groups, pain at multiple sites, fatigue, headache, depression, anxiety, paresthesia (numbness and tingling) and poor sleep patterns.

The condition is predominantly characterized by a consistent pattern of non-restorative or non-refreshing sleep–a sleep abnormality that is generally not a feature of other musculoskeletal diseases. A lack of refreshing sleep may be the major determining factor in the severity of FMS pain and cognitive impairments. It is, after all, sleep that allows damaged muscles and an over-stressed nervous system to recover, renew and regenerate. Studies indicate that anything done to improve sleep in victims of FMS improves, and in some cases even reverses, FMS altogether.

Sleep and the FMS Connection

Adequate sleep is an important component of good health, as it provides a time for the body to repair and replenish itself. Sleep deprivation or disturbed sleep cycles can lead to immune system imbalances such as those seen in fibromyalgia. And, indeed, a lack of non-restorative deep sleep is a prevailing characteristic of FMS.

Sleep occurs in cyclical patterns. In each typical sleep cycle of about ninety minutes the sleeper will spend three-quarters of the time in slow wave sleep (characterized by slow delta brain waves). The second stage is called D sleep, and although this is a deep sleep stage parts of the nervous system are very active. It is during this stage that rapid eye movements occur.

People with FMS have abnormalities in the slow wave stage of the normal sleep cycle. Importantly, it is this sleep stage that is thought to be physically restorative.

Referral to a sleep disorders clinic may be of some value to the 44 percent of men with FMS who also have obstructive sleep apnea, a potentially life-threatening disorder that requires treatment in its own right. In any resistant case of FMS, a sleep disorders clinic might also be helpful in evaluating sleep patterns and providing strategies to deal with altered sleep cycles.

9

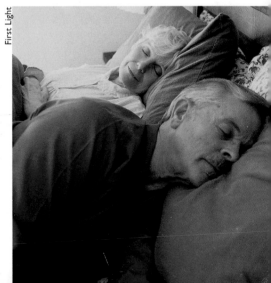

A lack of non-restorative deep sleep is a prevailing characteristic of Fibromyalgia.

In the past decade I have seen more than 1,000 patients who suffered from FMS. It is my experience that those patients who used some or all of the approaches outlined in this book made significant improvements. While no two people have the same combination of symptoms, and while the response to natural therapies is highly variable, people with FMS can indeed get better eventually. Health can be improved without dangerous drugs, as I will show in this book.

First Light

Signs and Symptoms . . . .

While there is no specific laboratory test that can diagnose FMS, conventional medicine currently defines the disease as a chronic, debilitating state of widespread musculoskeletal pain, stiffness and fatigue that meets at least the following criteria put forward by the American College of Rheumatology:

1) History of Widespread Pain
All of the following must be present:
- pain in the left side of the body
- pain in the right side of the body
- pain above and below the waist
- pain in either the spine, neck, front of the chest, thoracic spine or low back

2) Pain in 11 of 18 Tender Point Sites (on finger pressure)
- under the back of the skull
- lower neck muscles
- upper back muscles
- just above the bony protrusion in the back part of the shoulders
- second rib
- just below the elbow
- upper outer quadrant of buttock
- hip bone
- knee just proximal to the medial joint line

Common Fibromyalgia Symptoms . . . .

No two cases of FMS are identical with respect to the existence and/or severity of the symptoms. The percentages given for the conditions listed below are variable; they do, however, give an indication of the most predominate symptoms.

Conventional medicine offers no cure for FMS, just sleeping pills, antidepressants and other symptomatic drug treatments for pain control. But don't despair: This book describes a legitimate natural approach to reversing FMS based on the latest scientific studies and clinical observations of the top experts in the field.

Predominate Symptoms of Fibromyalgia

- Muscular pain, aching and/or stiffness, especially in the morning (100 percent)
- Badly disturbed sleep (nearly 100 percent)
- Symptoms worse in cold or humid weather (nearly 100 percent)
- History of injury within the year before the symptoms started (nearly 100 percent)
- Depression (70-100 percent depending on the study)
- Irritable bowel syndrome (34-73 percent)
- Severe migraine or non-migraine headaches (25-60 percent)
- Raynaud's phenomenon (numb fingers and toes 30-50 percent)
- Anxiety (24 percent)
- Sicca syndrome (dry eyes and/or mouth-18 percent)
- Osteoarthritis (12 percent)
- Rheumatoid arthritis (7 percent)

Other Common Conditions Associated with Fibromyalgia

- Allergies
- Digestive disturbances
- Dizziness
- Hair loss
- Flu-like illness symptoms (e.g., fever, swollen glands, headaches)
- Irritability
- Mood swings
- Night cramps
- Panic attacks
- Phobias
- Premenstrual syndrome
- Recurrent bladder sensitivity or infections
- Recurrent viral infections
- Short-term memory loss ("brain fog")
- Sleep apnea

It is important to first have a good understanding of exactly what is involved in FMS. Thus the material that follows will describe both the probable causes and the treatments that have, to date, been ignored by all but those knowledgeable in the natural healing arts.

What Causes Fibromyalgia? . . . .

Evidence is now accumulating that shows FMS is primarily a disorder of the immune system. The type of immune system disorder involved fits the category known as autoimmune disease.

An autoimmune disease is defined as one in which the body's immune system starts making antibodies against its own tissues or organs. In a normal state of health, the immune system recognizes the body's organs as native, or a part of self: It does not attack them in any way. A healthy immune system only attacks foreign invaders (e.g., bacteria, viruses, parasites) or tissues (cancer cells). When the immune system attacks normal healthy tissues and organs (self), it is defined as an autoimmune reaction.

An immune system reaction to joints (as in rheumatoid arthritis) is one example of an autoimmune reaction leading to an autoimmune disease. When the immune system mounts an attack against the thyroid, autoimmune thyroiditis results. When it attacks the lining of the gastrointestinal tract, autoimmune colitis (ulcerative colitis or Crohn's disease) results, and so on. Current thinking is that FMS is the result of such an autoimmune mechanism.

Immune System Reactions

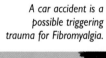

A car accident is a possible triggering trauma for Fibromyalgia.

The majority of FMS patients report that their chronic illness began with some definable traumatic trigger event—a severe flu-like illness that never really got better, for example. Alternatively, a motor vehicle accident that injured many different muscles, or a head injury that caused a loss of consciousness or a concussion may have been the triggering trauma. The trigger event was then followed by an abnormal or altered immune system reaction and the development of the signs and symptoms associated with FMS.

Autoimmunity in FMS victims is also evidenced by studies in which biopsies of muscles found edema (fluid

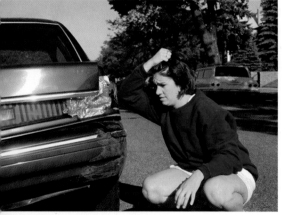

retention), elevated numbers of mast cells (cells involved in the allergic response), and increased fluid content—all suggestive of an allergic reaction of some sort.

Fibromyalgia syndrome is seen most often in those suffering from autoimmune disorders like rheumatoid arthritis, Raynaud's phenomenon and autoimmune thyroiditis (hypothyroidism). This observation lends further credibility to the idea that FMS is an autoimmune disorder since it is common for two or more autoimmune diseases to exist simultaneously in the same individual.

The Leaky Gut Connection

Autoimmune diseases have been linked to a general condition known as the leaky gut syndrome. A "leaky" gut is one in which the intestinal lining is more permeable than normal. In simple terms, this means that larger than optimal spaces are present between the cells of the gut wall, thereby allowing the entrance of bacteria, fungi, parasites, toxins, undigested protein, fat and waste material into the bloodstream. These substances, which are normally not absorbed in a healthy state, pass through a damaged, hyperpermeable or leaky gut.

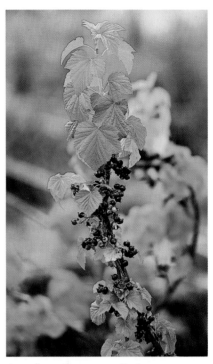

13

Black currants are rich in vitamin C and bioflavonoids, which help treat autoimmune diseases such as Fibromyalgia.

The leaky gut syndrome is brought about by inflammation of the gut lining. Inflammation causes the spaces between the cells to enlarge, allowing the absorption of large protein molecules. Normally these molecules would be broken down into much smaller pieces before absorption through the small spaces between the gut lining cells. The immune system starts making antibodies against the larger molecules because it recognizes these as foreign, invading substances. Thus antibodies are suddenly being made against the proteins and the previously well-tolerated foods.

These food antibodies can get into various tissues and trigger an inflammatory reaction when the corresponding food is consumed. This occurs because body tissues have antigenic sites very similar to those on food, bacteria, parasites, candida or fungi. Autoantibodies are thus created, and inflammation can become chronic. If this inflammation occurs in a joint, autoimmune arthritis develops. If it occurs in the blood vessels, vasculitis (inflammation of the blood vessels) is the resulting autoimmune problem. If it occurs in the muscles and multiple organ systems, the result may very well be FMS.

Leaky gut syndrome also creates a long list of mineral deficiencies because the various carrier proteins present in the gastrointestinal tract that are needed to transport minerals from the intestine to the blood are damaged by the inflammation process. For example, magnesium deficiency is quite a common finding in conditions like FMS despite a high magnesium intake through diet or supplementation. If the carrier protein for magnesium is damaged, magnesium deficiency develops as a result of malabsorption. Muscle pain and spasms can occur as a result.

Inflammation involves swelling (edema) and the presence of many noxious chemicals, all of which can block the absorption of vitamins and essential amino acids. A leaky gut does not absorb nutrients properly. Bloating, gas, cramping, and diarrhea alternating with constipation occur, leading to an irritable bowel syndrome. Eventually, systemic complaints like fatigue, headaches, memory loss, poor concentration or irritability develop.

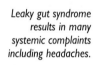

Leaky gut syndrome results in many systemic complaints including headaches.

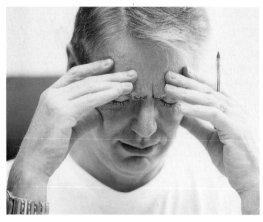

One of the major components of effective treatment of FMS involves a program of diet and nutritional supplements designed to repair the lining of the gastrointestinal tract and clear up the leaky gut phenomenon. A discussion of how one can both prevent and treat this condition is found in the treatment protocol section of this book.

The Mitochondrial Defect Connection

Fibromyalgia is also thought to be associated with sick mitochondria. Mitochondria are tiny cell organelles that basically

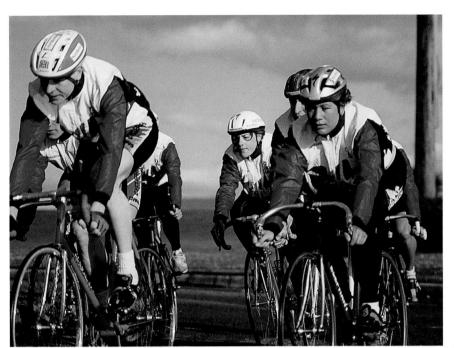

create energy to run the body. Physical fitness is, to a large degree, related to the number and health of the mitochondria. Elite athletes have higher numbers of healthy mitochondria in their cells than people who do not exercise.

Mitochondria can be damaged by viruses, bacteria, yeast toxins, chemicals, allergic reactions, excessive use of antibiotics and other prescription drugs, and toxic heavy metals like mercury, lead, cadmium and aluminum. The damaged mitochondria become the major source of free radicals, which eventually leads to a hyper-vigilant immune system that begins to react or attack the body's normal, healthy organs of the immune system (autoimmune reaction), resulting in an autoimmune condition like FMS.

People who suffer from FMS have damaged, suboptimal and inadequate levels of mitochondria in their cells. As a result, the biochemical processes that create energy function at a low rate, resulting in pain and fatigue. The good news is that sick mitochondria can be resuscitated through diet and nutritional supplements.

Elite athletes have a high number of healthy mitochondria, while sick mitochondria are associated with Fibromyalgia and low energy levels.

Substance P and Fibromyalgia

In early 1999, Dr. Laurence Bradley and his team of researchers from the University of Alabama discovered higher levels of a brain chemical called substance P in the cerebrospinal fluid of those with fibromyalgia. Higher levels of substance P have been linked to depression, poor concentration, pain, memory disturbance, and a hive-like reaction to a light scratching of the skin.

Substance P is a neurological chemical that allows cells in the nervous system to communicate with one another about potentially harmful stimuli. It is this chemical that transmits the signal that is interpreted by the brain as pain. According to Bradley, substance P levels are doubled or tripled in people with FMS, and can produce more episodes of pain transmission throughout the body. At present there are no direct and easy ways of controlling the levels of substance P. However, further research into substance P could eventually lead to a better understanding of the biochemical mechanisms seen in FMS, and thereby point to various treatments that could modulate these levels naturally.

Fibromyalgia Syndrome Treatment Protocol . . . .

Conventional medical treatments for FMS can only hope to keep symptoms under control; they pay no attention to the underlying source of the disorder. Only treatments aimed at the cause of the illness have any hope of eventually reversing FMS, and thus preventing it from becoming a lifelong condition.

A successful reversal of FMS involves the application of twelve different components of therapy. Each aspect of this treatment protocol is aimed at healing the immune, biochemical and hormonal defects that are at the root of the syndrome.

The FMS Diet

One's diet is, as always, an important variable in one's health, and is of particular importance to anyone suffering from a chronic illness like FMS. The best nutritional program to follow for those who suffer from FMS is a hypoallergenic diet. Ideally this is established on an individualized basis with the use of food allergy testing as well as other biochemical tests done through a natural health care provider. However, for those who can neither afford nor find such a doctor, the following is a basic hypoallergenic diet that I have used in my practice with a high degree of success. While it is radically different from the standard Canadian or American diet, it utilizes foods, which can, for the most part, be obtained from a supermarket, grocery or health food store.

This diet can be used by anyone suffering from candida (yeast-related illness), lactose intolerance, celiac disease and virtually any autoimmune disease including FMS, rheumatoid arthritis, lupus, scleroderma, ulcerative colitis and multiple sclerosis. The only caution is to avoid any foods that are known allergens. For example, if you are very allergic to apples, don't eat apples even though it is one of the foods allowed on the menus listed below. If you lose too much weight on this diet you are not getting enough calories. Just eat more of the allowed foods. If you have any doubts about any of the allowed foods, etc., consult a naturopath or medical doctor sympathetic to nutritional medicine.

Use organic foods whenever possible to avoid the deleterious effects of pesticides, hormones, antibiotics and genetically altered/engineered foods. I do not recommend the use of genetically altered/engineered foods simply because they have not been proven to be safe. If you do not already read food labels, now is the time to start. Avoid items containing hydrogenated saturated fats, modified vegetable oils, sugar and additives.

Avoid the effects of pesticides, hormones, antibiotics, and genetically engineered foods by eating organic produce.

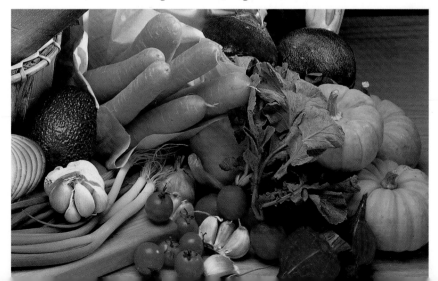

Allowed Foods and Beverages
(provided you are not allergic to them)

- Carotene-containing foods like sweet potatoes, carrots, spinach, cantaloupe, kale, squash, pumpkins and spinach These foods are excellent sources of beta carotene as well as other antioxidants.

- Rice cakes, rice cereals, rice bread and rice crackers. Rice is generally a very good alternative to wheat and provides many nutrients.

- Vitamin C- and antioxidant-containing foods like grapefruit, broccoli, strawberries, melons, Brussels sprouts and cabbages.

- Berries of all kinds, especially the European blueberry (a.k.a. bilberry), are rich in bioflavonoids. This strong antioxidant is known for its ability to resist free radical cell damage. Strawberries contain ellagic acid, a proven cancer-fighter that protects the body's genetic material from damage by carcinogens.

- Grapefruit provides a mighty force in protecting against allergies, inflammation, infection and cancer. Ruby red grapefruit is also a source of lycopene, an antioxidant similar to beta-carotene, which has potent cancer-fighting effects.

- Broccoli, Brussels sprouts and cabbages may not be your favorite foods but your body will love them. Along with relatives like kale, rutabaga and mustard greens, these vegetables help with liver detoxification. Broccoli may be the best of the bunch: One cup provides just 45 calories but has 4.5 grams of fiber and more than the recommended daily requirement of vitamin C and beta-carotene.

- Buckwheat, quinoa or rice pasta. These grain alternatives are very low in gluten and are generally better tolerated by people with disturbed immunity.

- All fresh fruits except lemons, limes, oranges and dried fruits (they are usually highly concentrated in fruit sugar).

- Lamb, poultry, fish and seafood. These foods are high in protein and are helpful in healing parasitic infestations. They must be well cooked.

- Organic fruit juices (freshly juiced) except for orange, lemon, lime and any sweetened juice. Citrus is a highly allergenic food containing citric acid, which can be a problem for highly sensitive people.

- Spring water, rice or almond milk. Rice and almond milk are good alternatives to milk.

- Small amounts of nuts. Avoid peanuts and cashews, which are contaminated with mold.

- Sunflower and pumpkin seeds. These are an excellent source of essential fatty acids and trace minerals such as zinc.

- Beans, lentils, dried peas, etc., are a rich source of protein, iron and calcium.

- Pure, filtered or ozonated water. It is important for adults to drink at least eight tall glasses of water every day.

The Elimination-Provocation Diet

Autoimmune diseases like FMS have been found to either reverse or improve when one eliminates common allergenic foods. While it would be more accurate to eliminate foods on the basis of food allergy testing, for those who can afford neither the time nor the money to get formal testing done, an elimination-provocation diet is a highly effective means of determining which foods one is allergic to.

Common Allergenic Foods

• Wheat and other gluten-containing grains (barley, oats, rye, spelt, amaranth, millet and kamut)

• Milk and dairy products

• Eggs

• Sugar in any form weakens the immune system and encourages the growth of bacteria, fungi, yeast and parasites. Stevia is a good alternative to sugar.

• Artificial sweeteners. Aspartame should be avoided at all cost since it has been found to worsen some of the mental/neurological signs and symptoms of FMS.

• Alcoholic beverages. Even "moderate" alcohol consumption is a problem since many with FMS have weak liver enzyme detoxification systems.

• Caffeine (coffee, regular tea, colas, chocolates). Caffeine interferes with sleep, which is an issue for those with FMS.

• Soft drinks

• Tap water (unless filtered by reverse osmosis or ozonated)

• All foods containing artificial flavorings, additives and preservatives,

• Beef, pork, cold cuts, fried foods and salty foods.

• Nightshade vegetables (tomatoes, potatoes, peppers, eggplants).

• Coconuts

• Peanuts, cashews and their products. (These products are all contaminated with mold and will worsen the symptoms of FMS.)

• Tropical fruit (bananas, pineapples, melons, papaya, mangoes, guava, passion fruit, kiwi). These fruits have a high sugar and mold content.

The basic concept behind this approach is to follow a hypoallergenic diet for three weeks, eliminating the most common food allergens, and thereafter challenging the body with the eliminated foods one by one, noting the reactions. During the three-week elimination diet, symptoms improve in the majority of people who suffer from food allergies. If the reintroduction of certain foods causes a reproduction of the symptoms, the person is probably allergic to those foods. This diet works only if all the foods to be discontinued are done so abruptly or "cold turkey." Easing into this diet slowly does not work nearly as well. Severely ill people should not try this approach without close supervision by a medical doctor. It is also advisable for anyone to seek the advice of a naturopath or doctor before beginning an elimination diet. (A detailed elimination diet is fully described in my book *Childhood Illness and The Allergy Connection* (Prima Books, 1996.)

Detection and Elimination of Allergies . . . . .

The signs and symptoms of all autoimmune disorders can be either reversed or significantly reduced in severity with the detection and elimination of allergic foods and chemicals. While these allergies are not necessarily the cause of the autoimmune condition, they most certainly can trigger flare-ups of symptoms or exacerbate existing symptoms such as pain, insomnia, fatigue and cognitive impairment.

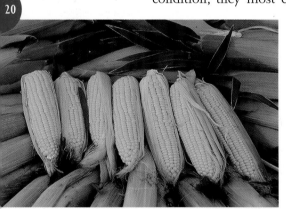

Food and chemical allergy testing is best done by means of an elimination-provocation diet. This is done by eliminating the most common allergenic foods (milk, dairy, wheat, gluten, citrus, corn, eggs, sugar, soy, beef, pork and yeast) for two to three weeks and then reintroducing them one by one, noting reactions.

Corn is one of the most common allergenic foods.

The majority of cases tested for food allergies show antibodies to gluten (from wheat) and/or casein (dairy protein), and benefit from a diet that eliminates dairy and all grains except rice, all refined carbohydrates, caffeine, red meats and processed foods. Nightshades foods (tomatoes, potatoes, peppers, eggplants, tobacco) might have to be eliminated by those who have joint pains associated with their consumption.

The majority of FMS victims do better if they give up caffeine, alcohol and other stimulants, as well as "excitotoxins" like monosodium glutamate (MSG), aspartame and hydrolyzed protein. Alcohol should definitely be avoided because of its tendency to suppress deep sleep. Carbonated beverages high in phosphates should also be eliminated since they can deplete calcium and magnesium from the body, two minerals FMS victims are usually deficient in.

The importance of giving up caffeine entirely cannot be stressed enough. For those with FMS, cutting down on caffeine doesn't just improve sleep; giving up caffeine also prevents low blood sugar levels, anxiety, irritability and the loss of trace minerals due to the diuretic effect of caffeine. It must be given up entirely.

The best way to get off the caffeine is to just stop. You may experience symptoms of caffeine withdrawal, including headache, fatigue and a craving for caffeine, but this only lasts a few days. Sleep often improves, along with many other FMS symptoms. Caffeine

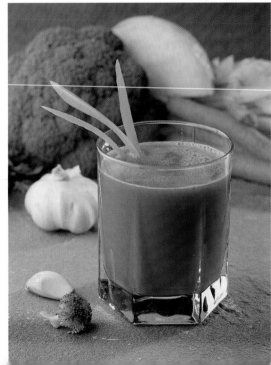

Those with Fibromyalgia must give up caffeine entirely. Vegetable juices are a healthful alternative.

is usually found in regular coffee, tea, chocolate, cola drinks (regular and diet varieties) and numerous over-the-counter and prescription analgesics.

Nutritional Supplements . . . .

While conventional medicine, such as antidepressants and sleeping pills, offer no cure for FMS, supplements work with the body to naturally prevent illness and restore health.

Essential Fatty Acids

Saturated animal fats and arachidonic acid (from red meats and dairy products) increase the inflammatory response by stimulating the production of the inflammatory prostaglandins and leukotrienes.

Prostaglandins are short-lived, hormone-like substances made by the body from essential fatty acids. They are produced in response to stimulatory events such as infection, trauma, allergy or toxin exposure. They regulate blood pressure, inflammatory responses, insulin sensitivity, immune responses, tissue building (anabolic) and tissue destroying (catabolic) processes, and hundreds of other biochemical reactions.

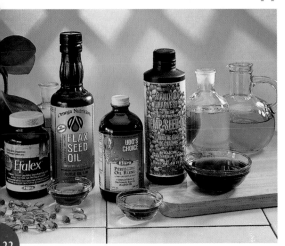

Supplementing with essential fatty acids promotes health and decreases inflammation.

The body makes both pro-inflammatory and anti-inflammatory prostaglandins depending upon the available amounts of various essential fatty acids obtained from the diet.

Prostaglandin E_1 is made from essential fatty acids and is anti-inflammatory. It prevents the creation of abnormal blood clots by inhibiting blood factors called platelets from aggregating, and promotes vasodilation and better circulation. Prostaglandin E_2, on the other hand, is generally produced from a diet too high in sugar, animal fats, hydrogenated or partially hydrogenated fats like vegetable shortening, margarine and refined oils, and junk foods. It promotes platelet aggregation, vasoconstriction, and is pro-inflammatory.

Supplementation with flax seed oil, evening primrose oil

and hempseed oil will ensure an adequate intake of the essential fatty acids that stimulate the synthesis of the anti-inflammatory prostaglandins that block the pain and inflammatory effects of chemical mediators like leukotriene.

An alternative way of obtaining anti-inflammatory essential fatty acids from the diet is to consume cold-water fish such as salmon, trout, mackerel, sardines, swordfish, shark, cod and halibut. These fish contain high concentrations of omega-3 fatty acids, which have also been documented to blunt the inflammatory or allergic response. If you find fish unpalatable or not readily available, supplementation with fish oil capsules is an alternative. Good vegetarian sources are flax seeds, walnuts, pecans, avocados, macadamia nuts, pumpkin seeds, sesame seeds and almonds.

Antioxidants

Antioxidants are enzymes, vitamins and minerals that prevent damage to cells and vital tissues in the body. In FMS, it is thought that mitochondrial injury in the cells is what causes the severe fatigue and muscle pain. Since the inflammatory response creates these sick mitochondria, the use of antioxidants helps prevent the damage that leads to permanent dysfunction. Antioxidant supplements include vitamins like carotenoids, beta-carotenes, vitamin A (retinol), bioflavonoids (rutin, hesperidin, quercetin, catechin), proanthocyanidins (grape seed extract, pine bark extract or pycnogenols), vitamins C and E, and sulfur-containing amino acids like cysteine, N-acetyl-cysteine, methionine and glutathione.

Supplementing with antioxidants helps to prevent the damage caused by Fibromyalgia.

Other important antioxidants with reported benefits for FMS are coenzyme Q10 and NADH, as well as B-complex vitamins (especially folic acid and vitamin B12), selenium and zinc. So-called superfoods like spirulina, chlorella, bee pollen, royal jelly and herbs of many different kinds have also been advocated. Whole-leaf aloe vera juice also contains high levels of dozens of natural antioxidants.

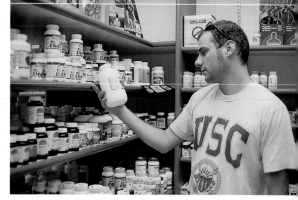

The nutrient coenzyme Q_{10} (CoQ_{10}) has been found to be very effective in treating FMS owing to the crucial role it plays in the production of energy in nearly every cell of the body. CoQ_{10} regulates the intake of oxygen into the mitochondria–the cell organelle thought to be damaged in FMS and other autoimmune diseases. Every cell in the body depends on CoQ_{10} to help turn food into energy. The recommended daily dose of this supplement is 100 to 200 mg, taken for at least two months. Some of the patients in my practice, as well as those of other nutritional doctors, find that relief from pain and increased energy levels only occurs with doses in the neighborhood of 400 to 600 mg of CoQ_{10} daily. My advice is to experiment with the low doses first and boost the dose if no effect is seen after six weeks.

The coenzyme NADH, which is present naturally in the body, has been found to boost energy levels in those with chronic fatigue syndrome, and may have the same effect on those with FMS. If cellular levels of NADH are depleted, brain and muscle cells lose their ability to function effectively. The theory is that as NADH levels rise in the body, the cells become more energized.

Magnesium and Malic Acid

There is some evidence for the therapeutic use of magnesium and malic acid in cases of FMS. Red cell magnesium levels are often low in those with FMS, and trial therapies with magnesium sulfate or magnesium chloride injections can be very effective. A magnesium deficiency can cause many of the symptoms of FMS, including fatigue, sleep disorders, mood disorders and muscle dysfunction.

Malic acid can be found in many fruits (especially apples) and vegetables and is also made in the body. It plays an important role in generating mitochondrial ATP, which is responsible for energy production. A lack of ATP causes muscle fatigue and pain.

The malic acid found in apples plays an important role in fighting the muscle fatigue and pain caused by Fibromyalgia.

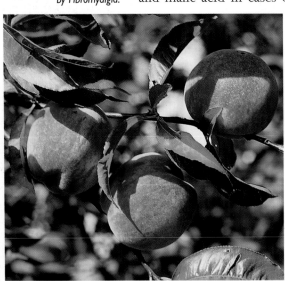

A study of twenty-four patients at the University of Texas Health Science Center in San Antonio treated with magnesium and malic acid showed reduced pain and tenderness after two months of supplementation. Recommended dosages are 150 mg magnesium and 600 mg malic acid twice a day with meals. Higher doses can be tried, but one should be careful with magnesium, as too much can cause diarrhea.

Amino Acids

S-adenosyl-methionine (SAM) is a derivative of the amino acid methionine, normally found in high-protein foods, especially animal products. Used extensively in Europe over the past twenty years, it has recently become popular as a treatment for depression, osteoarthritis and liver disorders. Some double-blind studies have shown it to offer symptom control for FMS as well. The only drawback to this remedy appears to be the price. The usual effective dose is 200 to 400 mg three times daily, and each 200 mg tablet costs between CAN $1.50 and $2.00. Given that SAM is a natural remedy not covered by Medicare or most drug plans, the cost may be affordable to only a handful of FMS victims.

The amino acid D,L-phenylalanine (DLPA) is found in high-protein foods, and is available as a food supplement without a prescription from most health food stores in the US. In Canada, it and other amino acid therapies can only be obtained with a prescription from a medical doctor. Several studies indicate that DLPA can be used to reduce pain and help with the depression that often accompanies FMS.

This supplement works by intensifying and prolonging the body's own natural pain-killing hormones, called endorphins, the substances that block pain signals moving through the nervous system. The body's endorphins have a narcotic-like effect when it comes to both the relief of pain and depression. Endorphins are released by intense physical activity, something not exactly in the repertoire of the average FMS

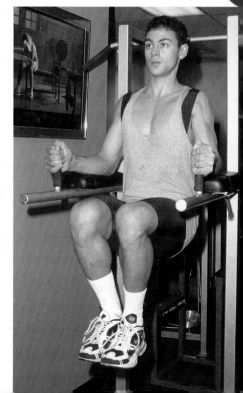

Amino acid supplements prolong the body's own natural pain-killing hormones. These hormones are released with intense physical activity, which is not always possible for someone with Fibromyalgia.

25

victim. Although DLPA is generally safe without adverse side effects, it should not be taken without consulting your health care practitioner.

The amino acid, L-carnitine is essential for energy production at the cellular level, especially in the heart and skeletal muscles. Carnitine is utilized to transfer fatty acids across the membranes of the mitochondria where they are used as a source of fuel to produce energy. Common symptoms of inadequate carnitine are fatigue and muscle pain. Many people with FMS can benefit from supplementing L-carnitine at doses of 1,000 mg twice daily. Again, this food supplement is not available in Canada but can be purchased in health food stores.

Hydrochloric Acid

Most autoimmune diseases are associated with a lack or insufficiency of hydrochloric acid production by the stomach. Achlorhydria (no acid) or hypochlohydria (low acid) leads to dozens of nutrient deficiencies. Most high-protein foods need acid for digestion. Amino acids, vitamins and minerals are poorly absorbed if acid is low or absent. The most recognized nutrient deficiency caused by low or deficient stomach acid is vitamin B_{12} deficiency, which leads to pernicious anemia and can usually only be rectified by regular vitamin B_{12} injections.

Low stomach acid may be the result of heredity, extended use of drugs (antacids, antiulcer medications), infection in the gut, or food allergies (especially to milk, dairy and wheat products).

Hydrochloric acid secretion, which aids in digestion, decreases with age.

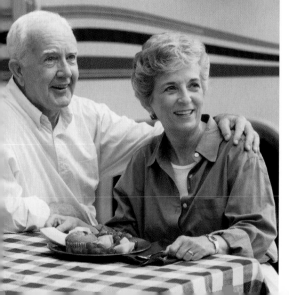

And hydrochloric acid secretion decreases with age. One study showed that by age sixty more than half the population has low stomach acidity. Low hydrochloric acid can be corrected by supplementing with stomach acidifiers like glutamic acid hydrochloride, betaine and pepsin hydrochloride, apple cider vinegar, lemon juice or stomach bitters. Also helpful in this respect are pantothenic acid (vitamin B_5), vitamin C, PABA and vitamin B_6.

Enzymes

Pancreatin (animal-based pancreatic digestive enzymes), plant enzymes and bromelain (from pineapples) not only help with protein digestion in the gastrointestinal tract but have been demonstrated to work as anti-inflammatory substances as well. They also help reduce the number of proinflammatory chemical mediators like some prostaglandins and leukotrienes.

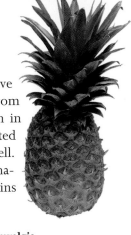

Nutritional supplements recommended for Fibromyalgia	
• Fish oil (or hempseed or flax oil):	9 to 12 grams daily
• Vitamin A:	10,000 IU daily
• Beta carotene:	20,000 IU daily
• Grape seed extract (pycnogenols):	300 mg daily
• B complex:	1 capsule 3 times daily
• Vitamin C:	1,000 mg 3 times daily
• Vitamin E:	800 IU daily
• Selenium:	200 mcg daily
• Zinc picolinate:	15 mg daily
• Copper citrate:	2 mg daily
• Coenzyme Q10:	100 to 600 mg daily
• N–acetyl–cysteine:	1,000 mg 3 times daily
• NADH:	2.5 mg twice daily
• Green drink (spirulina, chlorella, etc.):	1 tbsp daily
• Magnesium citrate:	500 mg daily
• Calcium citrate:	1,000 mg daily
• Malic acid:	1,000 mg 3 times daily

Herbs

Curcumin: The yellow pigment of the herb tumeric is called curcumin. In some studies it has been reported to be as effective as cortisone without any of the associated side effects. Curcumin is primarily effective as a natural anti-inflammatory agent but it also has important uses in cancer prevention, liver disorders, heart disease and irritable bowel syndrome. In fibromyalgia, as in most other autoimmune disorders, curcumin is most effective as an antioxidant as well as to support liver detoxification enzyme systems. Patients using it report less pain and higher energy levels.

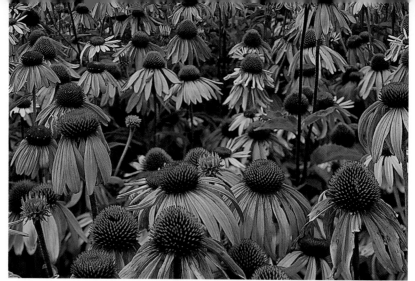

The immune-boosting and anti-inflammatory effects of echinacea play an important role in treating Fibromyalgia and other autoimmune diseases.

Echinacea: Echinacea is a very popular North American herb used to treat a variety of symptoms and diseases. It has anti-inflammatory properties, and as such it has a valid and often very effective role to play in all autoimmune diseases. High doses of echinacea for extended periods of time can reduce pain just about anywhere. Contrary to popular belief, there is no evidence to suggest that the use of echinacea should be interrupted for several weeks at a time. In fact, for those with FMS, long-term daily use is desirable.

Ginger: This herb is not only a good treatment for nausea and motion sickness but has a natural anti-inflammatory effect in arthritis, bursitis and other musculoskeletal ailments. Since over 70 percent of FMS victims have some degree of gastrointestinal tract irritability, ginger is an excellent choice for daily use.

Black Cohosh: *Cimicifuga* has traditionally been used for pain, muscular spasms, and muscular and uterine inflammatory conditions, and is thus useful for FMS. Black cohosh roots contain the anti-inflammatory salicin, which helps alleviate muscle and joint pain.

Calendula: Also known as marigold, this is a herb with a wide range of applications. It can be taken as a tincture or brewed as a tea. Although not generally discussed as a therapy for fibromyalgia, calendula can have remarkably good results in reversing both pain and fatigue in FMS. This is most likely due to its antiviral and antimicrobial effects, but this has not yet been verified by any specific studies.

St. John's Wort (hypericum): This popular herb is an effective mild to moderate antidepressant, analgesic and sedative. Effective doses of St. John's Wort are 2 to 4 grams of the raw herb or 0.2 to 1.0 mg of extracted hypericin (the purported active ingredient) per day. Common antidepressant dosage is 300 mg three times daily and before bedtime. Some of my patients have been successful in keeping off more toxic psychiatric drugs by taking doses of the herb at levels of 600 mg four times daily for several years on end.

Ginkgo: "No ginkgo, no thinko" is an expression coined by my older son, Mattie, who has, no doubt, attended far too many of my lectures on the use of ginkgo for memory enhancement. The fact is that victims of FMS often report a problem with brain fog, forgetfulness, difficulty with short-term memory and a general feeling of "spaciness." Ginkgo biloba extract is very effective in reversing all these symptoms at doses ranging from 250 to 500 mg daily. Ginkgo biloba has traditionally been used to improve memory and mental function and reduce the symp-

Ginkgo biloba extract is very effective in reversing symptoms related to memory, concentration and circulation.

toms of inadequate circulation to the brain. It enhances the flow of blood, carrying vital oxygen and glucose to the brain while acting as a free radical scavenger. It basically helps clear the cobwebs. Ginkgo improves concentration, possibly by increasing the rate at which information is transmitted between nerve cells.

Kava: Kava is an inexpensive herb used to ease anxiety without significant side effects. Kava can be taken during the day since it is non-sedating and is helpful in breaking the cycle of pain/ stress/more pain. Suggested dosage is 250 to 1,000 mg taken three times a day with food. Look for standardized extracts with at least 30 percent kavalactones, the purported active ingredient.

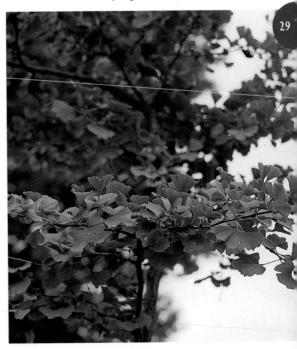

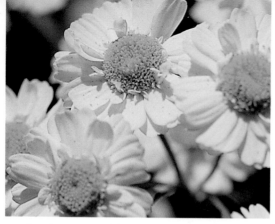

Herbs such as comfrey, white willow bark, feverfew, devil's claw, yarrow, yucca and marshmallow may also be helpful natural anti-inflammatory agents. And tea tree oil can be a very effective muscle pain reliever when applied and gently massaged into sore or weak muscles on a regular basis.

Feverfew is a natural anti-inflammatory agent.

Antifungal Regimes and Probiotics . . . .

Autoimmune diseases often respond to antifungal treatments. Evidence exists that fungi, through their production of myco-toxins, initiate many autoimmune diseases by triggering inflammation in the gastrointestinal tract, which in turn leads to the development of the leaky gut syndrome. Diseases of "unknown etiology" often have a fungal connection, with treatment of the fungal infection bringing about an improvement or elimination of that disease.

In treating any fungal infection, it is important to realize that many foods, even those considered to be healthy, are heavily colonized by fungi and their mycotoxins. These include corn, peanuts, cashews and dried coconuts. To a lesser degree, fungi can also be found in barley, rye, wheat, rice, millet and practically all cereal grains. A diet high in contaminated grains and nuts increases the likelihood of fungal colonization of the gastrointestinal tract. Worse, animals fed mycotoxin-contaminated

Many foods increase the likelihood of fungal colonization in the gastrointestinal tract.

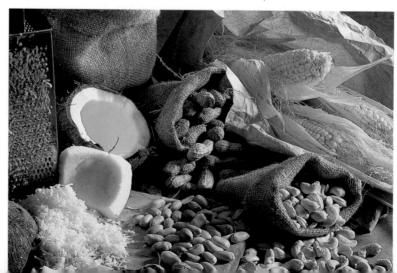

grains end up with fungal overgrowth. This is evidenced by the fact that the fat and muscles of most grain-fed animals in North America are loaded with mycotoxins. While it cannot be said that fungi and their mycotoxins cause FMS, there are numerous reports that the use of antifungal remedies clears or improves many cases of this condition.

Hormonal Therapies . . . .

Fibromyalgia syndrome and other autoimmune diseases have been reported to respond in varying degrees to low doses of DHEA, pregnenolone, cortisol, estrogen, progesterone, testosterone and thyroid hormones.

In Fibromyalgia, there is significant stress on the adrenal, gonadal and thyroid glands.

In FMS, there is significant stress on the adrenal, gonadal and thyroid glands. There are numerous reports that people with fibromyalgia have lower than optimal levels of the hormones associated with these glands, such as thyroid hormone T3, DHEA, testosterone, cortisol and progesterone. Providing these hormones as a supplement often improves or even clears FMS problems. However, before trying hormonal remedies, hormone levels should first be established through lab tests and consultation with your health care practitioner.

Women are affected by fibromyalgia anywhere from eight to twenty times more often than men. It is thought that hormones play a part in this differentiation. In fact, evidence exists that supplementing either men or women with male hormones like testosterone and DHEA will improve or even eliminate the numerous signs and symptoms of FMS.

Androgens (male hormones) are produced by the adrenal cortex of both males and females, and DHEA is the most abundant of these male hormones. It can be found in almost any organ, including the testes, the ovaries, the lungs and the brain. Testosterone is synthesized from DHEA in both males and females. One of the theories as to why females get autoimmune diseases at a much higher rate than males is that the relatively higher levels of DHEA and testosterone in males provide some sort of defense against such illnesses. Male hormones are muscle-building and energy-enhancing; they also have an anti-inflammatory, antiallergy effect.

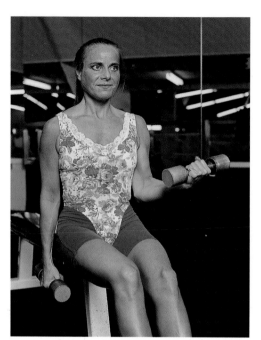

Fibromyalgia affects women eight to twenty times more often than men.

These characteristics may be significant in avoiding conditions like FMS. Natural precursors to DHEA can be found in wild yam, but studies do not indicate that this is equivalent to the pure hormone. Testosterone can be used if DHEA fails to produce positive results. The dose for DHEA is 5 to 25 mg for women, and 5 to 50 mg for men, but it depends on levels determined by lab test. For testosterone, the dosages would be roughly the same. In Canada, these hormones must be prescribed by a doctor; in the United States, these hormones are available without a prescription.

An alternative to testosterone itself is velvet elk antler, a natural product containing precursors to testosterone. Velvet elk antler has been used as a nutritional supplement in China for over 2,000 years, and is as important in traditional Chinese medicine as ginseng. Velvet elk antler is a renewable resource harvested humanely each year from specially bred elk during the rapid growth phase of antler. It is purported to boost energy and enhance immunity and has recently caught the attention of North Americans interested in better health and longevity.

Caution: Although no significant side effects have been reported with velvet elk antler, check with your doctor before self-administering, especially if you are currently being treated for a medical condition.

Thyroid Hormones

There is a school of thought that FMS is the result of low levels of T3, one of the thyroid hormones associated with thyroid regulation. According to alternative health care doctors, underarm temperatures of 97.6° F or below (or average oral temperatures below 98.6° F) on a regular basis combined with symptoms of low metabolism are likely due to a hidden hypothyroid (low thyroid) condition.

The classic symptoms of a low functioning thyroid include many of those associated with FMS: depression, fatigue, cold extremities, fluid retention, trouble losing weight, a higher than average body fat composition, heart beat irregularities, gastrointestinal symptoms such as multiple food sensitivities/allergies, and poor response to exercise (e.g., getting weaker after months of aerobic exercising). Temperature checking for low thyroid is best done using an old-fashioned shake-down thermometer. Taking daily readings for a few weeks will show an accurate trend.

Low temperatures may also be a reflection of suboptimal nutrient levels in the body. Consequently, nutritional factors must also be considered, and include deficiencies in protein, zinc, selenium, silicon, iodine (sea kelp), vitamin A, B-complex vitamins (particularly biotin and inositol), essential fatty acids, vitamin C and vitamin E. Routine blood tests for thyroid may be normal in unsuspected ("subclinical") hypothyroidism. One may, however, find a higher than normal cholesterol, and a low vitamin A and high carotene level. This phenomenon occurs because active thyroid hormone is required to convert carotene from the diet into vitamin A (retinol). It is also required to help keep cholesterol blood levels low.

Low body temperature may be an indication of a hidden hypothyroid condition or of suboptimal nutrient levels.

33

In most cases of hypothyroidism, especially in vegetarians, vitamin A will be low while carotene will be high on the blood tests. Evidence of this is a carrot-orange color on the palms and soles. Many people who have normal thyroid function tests with multiple hypothyroid symptoms will occasionally show high levels of antithyroid antibodies and antimicrosomal antibodies (Hashimoto's Thyroiditis). The B vitamin PABA, high doses of primrose oil or other essential fatty acids, and vitamin E in high doses may then be very helpful to reverse the condition. If not, low doses of prescribed thyroid hormone (i.e., desiccated thyroid), slow-release liothyronine (T3), glandular thyroid extract or homeopathic thyroid drops may help relieve symptoms.

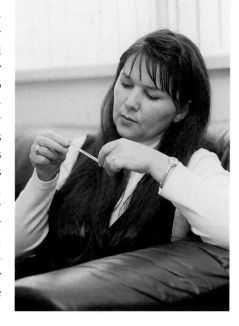

Removal of Mercury Amalgam

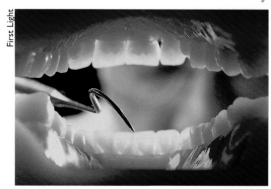

First Light

The mercury in dental fillings may be linked to Fibromyalgia.

In many cases of autoimmune disease, replacement of mercury with non-metal fillings is effective at reversing symptoms. Mercury may well be behind the immune system abnormalities leading to conditions like fibromyalgia.

Despite the fact that over 100 published scientific papers directly implicate mercury released from amalgam restorations as a major contributing factor in chronic illness, groups like the Canadian Dental Association (CDA) refuse to acknowledge this. It should be noted that no government or professional agency has ever shown that mercury in dental amalgams is safe.

Mercury can indirectly increase antibiotic-resistant oral and intestinal bacteria, impair kidney function and induce autoimmune diseases like FMS, multiple sclerosis and chronic fatigue syndrome. Several neurological diseases are linked to mercury hypersensitivity or toxicity including Lou Gehrig's disease, Parkinson's disease and Alzheimer's disease.

A growing number of dentists are ignoring the irresponsible edicts of dental associations and have decided to work without mercury for the protection of themselves and their patients. Mercury is a toxic substance in any amount. It does not belong in your mouth. Find a dentist that acknowledges this fact and

34

works without mercury. Inert non-metal composite or porcelain fillings are a much safer (and more attractive) alternative.

It must be stressed that the removal and replacement of amalgam fillings releases mercury vapors and can worsen symptoms, especially in highly sensitive individuals like those suffering from FMS. Such individuals should consult a natural health care practitioner or medical specialist before replacing mercury fillings.

To prevent or offset mercury damage from the replacement of dental amalgams, one can follow a high fiber diet, eat more garlic and onions, drink distilled water and supplement with high doses of beta-carotene, vitamin A, vitamin C, selenium, vitamin E, aloe vera juice, green drinks like barley green, chlorella, spirulina, blue green algae and sulfur-containing amino acids like cysteine, methionine, N-acetyl-cysteine and glutathione. This regimen is also acceptable as a way of preventing free radical damage to the body by any toxic heavy metal including mercury. (To find a dentist in your area who knows about mercury alternatives, see the "Sources" on page 62).

Exercise

Studies have shown that aerobic exercise (swimming, walking) improves muscle fitness and reduces muscle pain and tenderness. Daily gentle, low-impact aerobic exercise or water exercise has been validated as effective FMS therapy for a small number of cases in controlled trials; this is most likely because exercise increases the time spent in deep sleep. Start out with three to five minutes of exercise every day and increase as tolerated up to twenty or thirty minutes a day. Exercise works best if one avoids exercising the most painful muscles. One must be careful not to overdo physical activity because this may trigger a relapse.

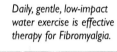

Daily, gentle, low-impact water exercise is effective therapy for Fibromyalgia.

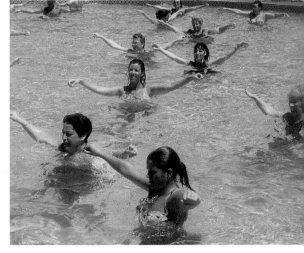

Exercise and Fibromyalgia

Because of the pain associated with fibromyalgia, many of those suffering with this condition have curtailed their physical activity and no longer get adequate amounts of exercise. Over time muscles become weak, and ligaments and tendons are more prone to injury. It is important, therefore, to get as much exercise as one can possibly endure, even if it is just a few minutes a day. Given that the symptoms of fibromyalgia vary considerably among individuals, it is impossible to outline an exercise strategy suitable for all those with FMS. I would recommend that one consult a physiotherapist or health practitioner and work with him or her to design an exercise program that will provide stretching, strengthening and aerobic activity that suits your abilities. You will not only feel better physically but mentally as well.

Physical Therapies

Acupuncture, cranio-sacral therapy, massage therapy, hydrotherapy, osteopathy and Reiki are just a few of the many physical ("hands on") therapies that have been reported to help FMS. While not everyone responds equally well, or sometimes at all, from any of these treatment modalities, they are at least worth trying as alternatives to drugs for pain control and sleep enhancement. In addition, self-help treatments like meditation, relaxation and yoga can better control stress and prevent relapses after gains are made from various diet and lifestyle adjustments.

Consider using magnetic therapies as well. The body normally has an electric field that can be affected by electromagnetic forces, both to its benefit and detriment. People who suffer from pain of any kind, regardless of whether they have FMS, can be helped by magnetic therapy. Specifically designed magnets can be applied directly to areas of pain or discomfort, especially after exercise or physical exertion, or they may be worn during the day when pain tends to be most severe. Magnetic therapy has been documented to enhance circulation, increase oxygen flow and bring needed nutrients to the area of pain. Pregnant women or those wearing implanted medical devices such as pacemakers or insulin pumps should not use magnets.

Reflexology, especially on the reflexes corresponding to the kidneys, liver, adrenal glands and solar plexis, is an effective treatment for Fibromyalgia.

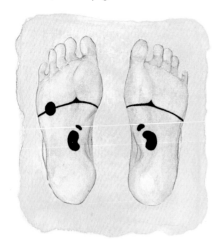

Controlled studies have shown that EMG biofeedback, regional sympathetic blockade and cognitive behavioral therapy are also helpful in cases of fibromyalgia. EMG biofeedback is an electronic pain relief therapy and is available from a physiotherapist, physiatrist or chiropractor. Regional sympathetic blockade involves the injection of an anesthetic into the spinal cord for analgesia. It is usually provided by an MD or anesthetist. Cognitive behavioral therapy is a type of short-term, behavior-based psychotherapy. All these therapies can help with some or all the symptoms of FMS.

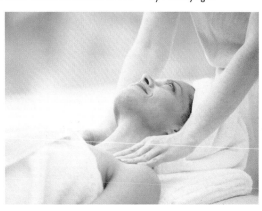

Regular, gentle massage helps relieve pain caused by Fibromyalgia.

Intravenous Therapies . . . .

Many physicians have had success in reversing the signs and symptoms of FMS using an intravenous vitamin and mineral protocol known as "Myers' Cocktail." This consists of the following:

Magnesium chloride hexahydrate (20 percent): 2-5 ml
Calcium gluconate (10 percent): 2-4 ml
Hydroxocobalamin (vitamin B12): 1,000 mcg/ml-1 ml
Pyridoxine hydrochloride: 100 mg/ml-1 ml
Dexpanthenol (vitamin B5): 250 mg/ml-1 ml
B complex: 100 mg/ml-1 ml
Vitamin C: 222 mg/ml

This mixture is combined with sterile water and is injected intravenously over a period of five to fifteen minutes. Improvements in symptoms are noticeable from within minutes to hours of the injection, and the procedure can be repeated as often as needed to reverse FMS. Side effects are rare to non-existent. Typically, the patient that responds to this therapy does so after a series of a dozen or more IVs over a period of several months. The Myers' cocktail should be considered as a treatment option, especially by those who get little to no benefit from diet modification or oral supplements, as well as by those who have trouble swallowing numerous pills. Obviously, this is a therapy that can only be provided by a doctor or naturopath.

Rebalancing Neurotransmitters . . . .

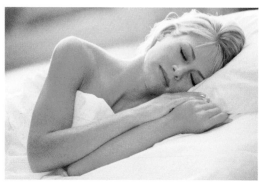

L-tryptophan, a precursor to serotonin, can be used to improve sleep instead of the psychoactive drugs commonly prescribed.

Some studies have shown that levels of serotonin and its dietary precursor tryptophan are low in those with FMS. Serotonin is a neurotransmitter that is released in the synapse between two nerve cells. Once released, some of the serotonin goes to transmit a message to the other cell to relax and some of it is taken back by the cell that released the serotonin in the first place. This latter activity is called reuptake. If one inhibits this reuptake, more serotonin is available in the synapse and one gets more of the benefits of serotonin, which includes deep sleep. Thus supplements that inhibit reuptake of seratonin can increase deep sleep, which is of primary importance for those with FMS. Tryptophan is a precursor to serotonin and can be used for sleep improvement in place of the psychoactive drugs so commonly prescribed for people with FMS.

Another way of balancing neurotransmitters is to supplement with melatonin (1 to 3 mg before bedtime). While not effective in every case of FMS, there is good scientific evidence for its use in treating sleep disorders of any kind. Melatonin is a hormone secreted by the pineal gland (part of the brain stem), mainly at night. Its primary role is that of an antioxidant, protecting our tissues from daily damage by harmful chemicals and other toxins. Because melatonin helps improve sleep and works as an effective antioxidant, it is logical and quite correct to assume that it will also help a large number of FMS symptoms associated with poor sleep patterns and oxidant damage to the mitochondria.

Given these facts, why has the Canadian Health Protection Branch (HPB) ordered melatonin off the shelves? The answer is fairly simple: The HPB reacts to the whim and desires of its true masters, the multinational drug companies. Melatonin administration raises brain serotonin levels. Conversely, when serotonin levels are increased, so is melatonin. The new generation of very profitable antidepressants (Prozac® and Zoloft® among others) have the same effect. These drugs are currently estimated to be taken by over 40 million people in North America for depression, insomnia, obsessive compulsive disorders, eating disorders, anxiety, premenstrual syndrome and general stress reduction. Many who suffer from FMS take one or more of these mood-altering drugs. At roughly three dollars or more a pill, do the drug companies that market them really want a competitor that sells the same effect for less than twenty-five cents a pill in the form of melatonin?

Fibromyalgia is a reversible condition without the need for prescription medications.

There is Hope . . . .

Fibromyalgia syndrome is a reversible condition, and the majority of those who use the protocols outlined in this book will regain their health and the lives they once led—without the need for prescription medications. The time frame for recovery varies from person to person but all can expect to see some improvement in their symptoms in three to five weeks. A full recovery for most may take from six to twelve months, with those under the age of forty-five having the quickest response to natural therapies. Although it is true that the majority of the twelve steps of the FMS protocol can be done without the need to consult a physician, results could be enhanced with regular consultations with a naturopath or medical doctor familiar with a natural approach.

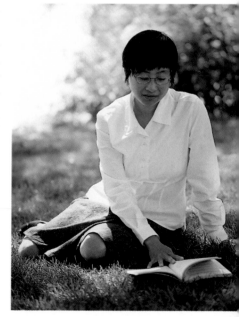

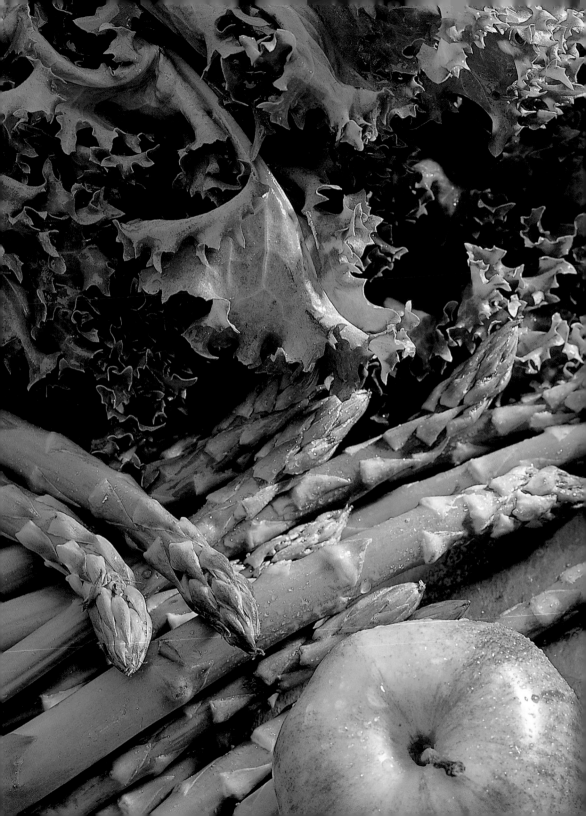

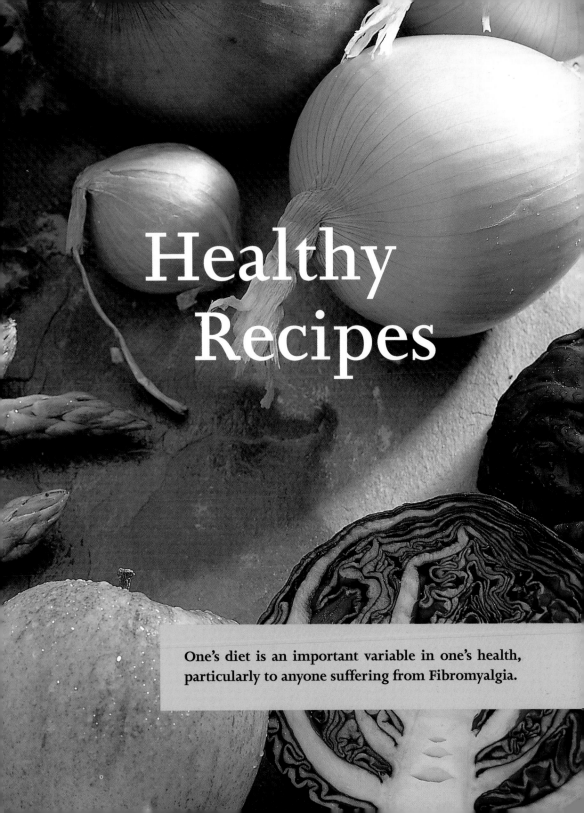

Healthy Recipes

One's diet is an important variable in one's health, particularly to anyone suffering from Fibromyalgia.

Cream of Rice Cereal with Fresh Fruit

There's no reason to get bored with rice, as long as you have tasty, whole food recipes. After all, Asians around the world enjoy rice every day without getting bored with it. It is a good alternative to wheat and can be safely eaten by gluten-intolerant people.

1 cup (250 ml) rice meal

1½ cups (375 ml) distilled or filtered water

¼ cup (60 ml) rice or almond milk

1 tsp vanilla extract

1 tbsp cold-pressed flax seed oil

1 cup (250 ml) strawberries, quartered

1 cup (250 ml) blueberries

1 cup (250 ml) red or white grapes

In a pot, cook rice in water on low heat, stirring continuously, until thick and all water is absorbed. Stir in rice milk, vanilla extract and flax seed oil, making sure cereal is not too hot. Pour into bowls, add fruit and serve.

Serves 2

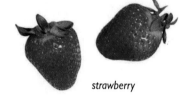

strawberry

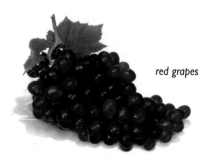

red grapes

It's easy to make homemade almond milk out of soaked almonds and pure water. For recipes, see Nomi Shannon's classic raw foods book, *The Raw Gourmet* (alive books, 1999).

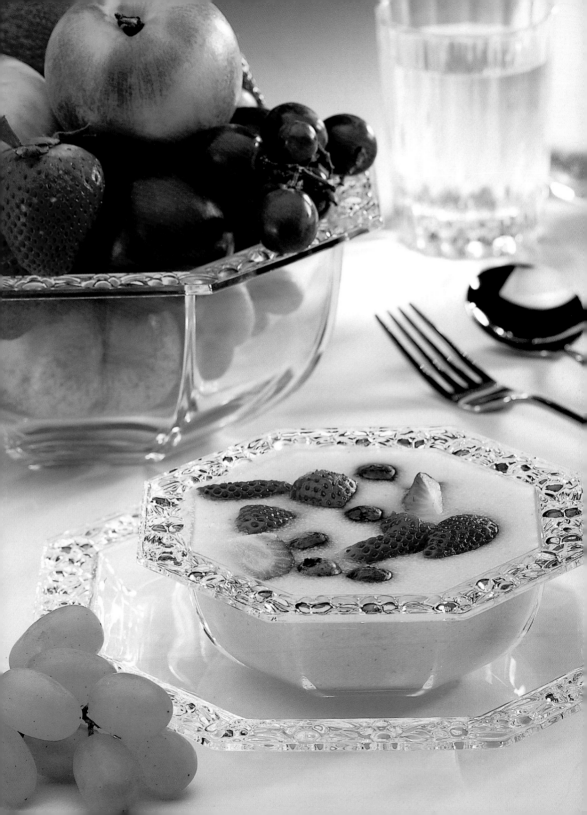

Creamy Cauliflower-Spinach Soup with Roasted Garlic

This soup won't make you deviate from the recommended Fibromyalgia diet, since it's cauliflower–not cream–that give it the creaminess.

1 whole bulb garlic

2 tbsp + 2 tbsp extra-virgin olive oil

Sea salt and freshly ground pepper, to taste

1 tsp dried thyme

1 cup (250 ml) white onion, diced

3 cloves garlic, minced

1 cup (250 ml) cauliflower, cut in chunks

1 cup (250 ml) parsnips, cut in chunks

1 qt (1 L) vegetable stock

1 bay leaf

2 cups (500 ml) spinach, chopped

1 tbsp cold-pressed almond oil

Preheat oven to 375°F (190°C).

To roast the garlic, cut the top off the garlic bulb so that the cloves are just showing. In an ovenproof pan, brush the bulb with 2 tablespoons of olive oil and season with salt, pepper and thyme. Place on the top shelf of the oven and bake for 35 to 40 minutes or until garlic is golden brown.

In the meantime, heat 2 tablespoons of oil in a large pot over medium heat and sauté onion and minced garlic until tender. Add cauliflower, parsnips, vegetable stock, bay leaf and season with salt and pepper.

Cover and cook on medium heat for 20 to 25 minutes or until vegetables are tender. Remove soup from heat and remove bay leaf. Pour soup into blender, add spinach and blend until smooth. Return to pot and warm.

Drizzle with almond oil and serve with roasted garlic.

Serves 2

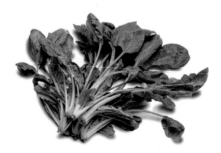

spinach

44

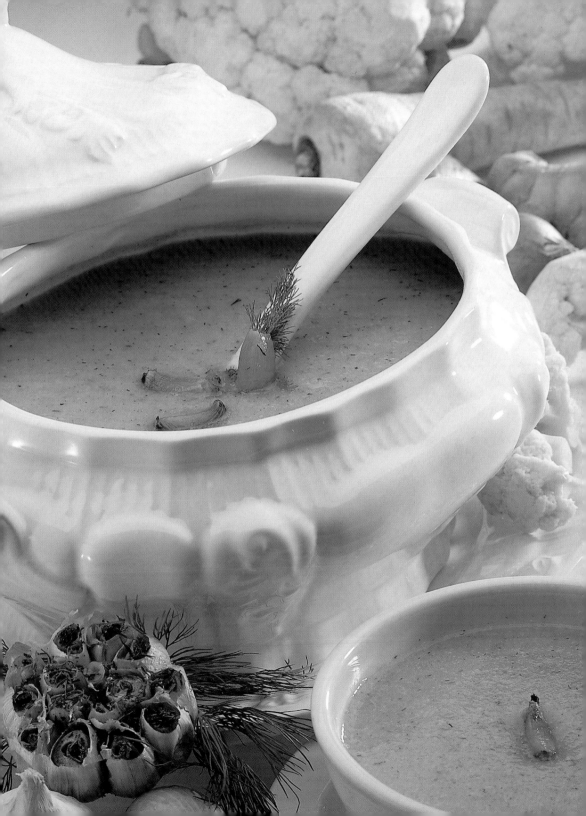

Waldorf Salad with Watercress

This lively combination of radish and watercress with a unique dressing gives a greater bite than traditional Waldorf salads. Watercress is a hardy plant that supplies twice the calcium of broccoli and just as much vitamin A as carrots.

1 cup (250 ml) **red radish, cut in ¼" (5 mm) strips**

1 cup (250 ml) **apple, cut in ¼" (5 mm) strips**

1 cup (250 ml) **celery root, cut in ¼" (5 mm) strips**

¼ cup (60 ml) **toasted walnuts**

2 cups (500 ml) **watercress**

Dressing:

4 tbsp **cold-pressed walnut oil**

2 tbsp **freshly pressed grape juice**

2 tsp **tahini**

1 tsp **fresh mint, chopped**

In a large bowl, whisk together all dressing ingredients. Toss radish, apple, celery and walnut with half the dressing.

Place watercress onto plates, drizzle with remaining dressing and arrange vegetables over top.

Serves 2

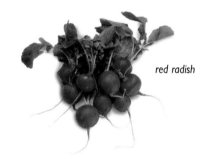

red radish

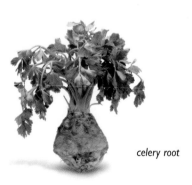

celery root

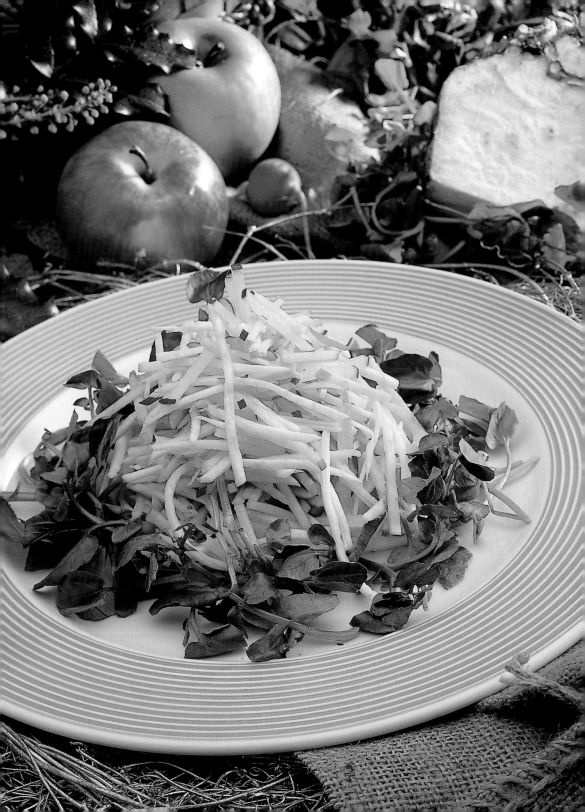

Cucumber-Fennel Salad

Fennel, or finnochio, as the Italians call it, imparts a sweet delicate flavor to this salad. It's high in vitamin A, so combined with carrots, this dish will give you plenty of protective antioxidants.

I large English cucumber, sliced

I cup (250 ml) radish, sliced

I cup (250 ml) fennel bulb, julienned

I cup (250 ml) carrots, julienned

Fresh parsley, for garnish

Dressing:

¼ cup (60 ml) freshly pressed apple juice

2 tbsp freshly pressed carrot juice

2 tbsp cold-pressed flax seed oil

I tbsp extra-virgin olive oil

In a large bowl, whisk together all dressing ingredients then toss with cucumber, radish, fennel and carrots.

Place salad onto plates, garnish with parsley and serve.

Serves 2

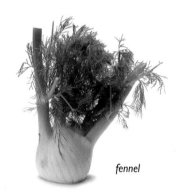

fennel

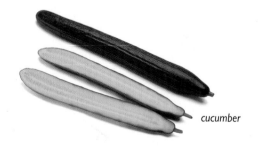

cucumber

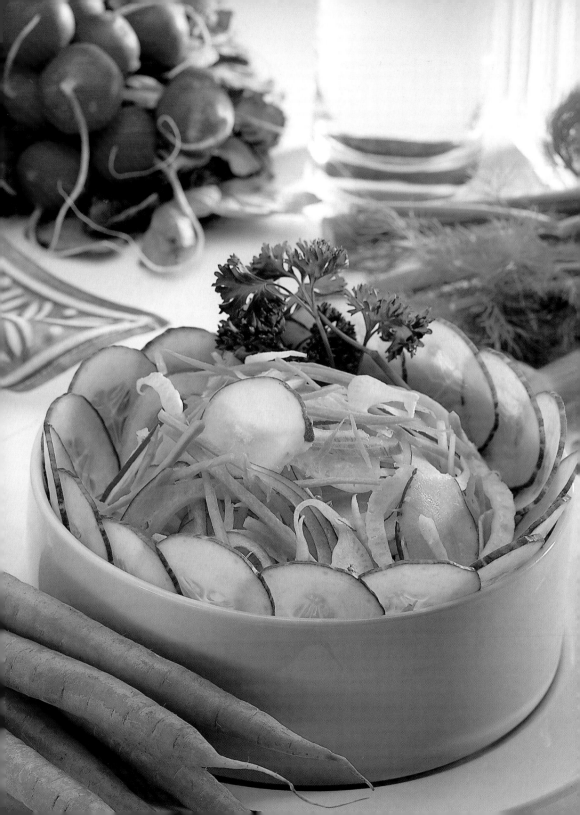

Warm Asparagus-Avocado-Zucchini Salad

A delicacy from ancient times, asparagus is a good source of the antioxidant vitamins A, C and E, as well as the minerals potassium and zinc.

1 lb (500 g) asparagus, trimmed and cut in 3" (7.5 cm) pieces

1 large carrot, peeled and shaved lengthwise (thinly sliced)

1 large zucchini, shaved lengthwise

1 ripe avocado, cut in wedges

Dressing:

2 tsp tahini

1 tbsp green onion, chopped

1 tbsp tamari

1 tsp Dijon mustard

¼ cup (60 ml) cold-pressed flax seed oil

Blanch asparagus for 3 minutes in a pot of boiling salted water. Drain and immediately rinse with cold water. Set aside.

In a bowl, whisk together all dressing ingredients. Pour in a pan and heat on low until just warm.

Place vegetables in a bowl and toss with the warm dressing. Place onto plates and serve.

Serves 2

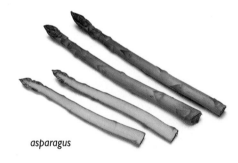

asparagus

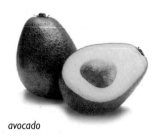

avocado

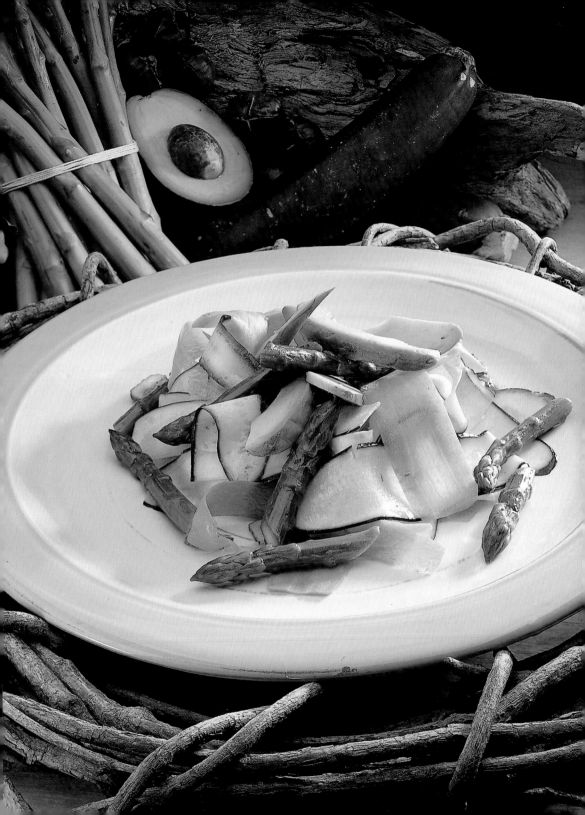

Apple-Green Bean Salad

Besides providing enzymes, minerals and protein, this fantastic combination of fresh apple and green beans will amaze and delight your taste buds. That's why I serve it as a whole meal–it'll satisfy you completely.

1 cup (250 ml) **green beans**

2 cups (500 ml) **apple, cut in chunks**

2 cups (500 ml) **carrot, julienned**

½ cup (125 ml) **red onion, diced**

4 tbsp cold-pressed hazelnut or walnut oil

2 tbsp fresh grape juice

Herbamare seasoning, to taste

Blanch beans in a pot of boiling salted water for 2 to 3 minutes. Drain and immediately rinse under cold water.

In a bowl, whisk together oil and juice. Season with salt and pepper. Add beans, apple, carrot and onion and toss thoroughly.

Serves 2

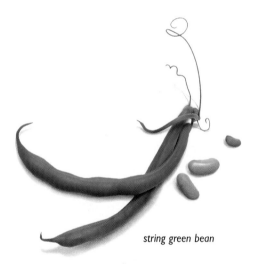

string green bean

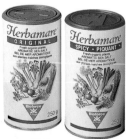

Herbamare

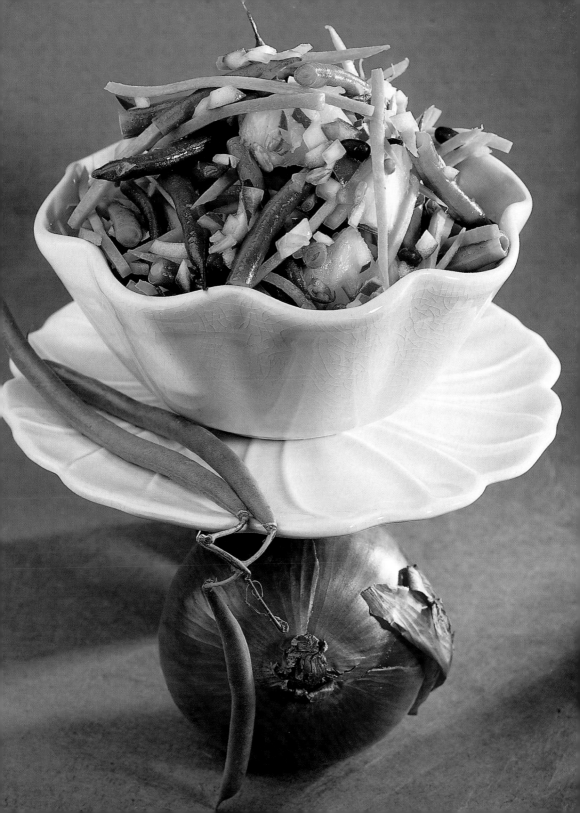

Vegetable Spring Roll with Yam

These spring rolls, made with rice flour wraps and stuffed with carotene-rich vegetables, are a delightful variation on the traditional Asian specialty.

2 medium yams, peeled and cut 3" (7.5 cm) long and ½" (1 cm) wide

2 tbsp extra-virgin olive oil

2 tbsp onion, chopped

1 tsp garlic, minced

1 tsp ginger, minced

1 cup (250 ml) carrots, julienned

1 cup (250 ml) fennel root, julienned

1 cup (250 ml) turnip, julienned

1 cup (250 ml) zucchini, julienned

1 cup (250 ml) leeks, julienned

1 tsp cilantro, chopped

4 pieces rice paper

Bring a pot of salted water to a boil and blanch yam for 7 to 10 minutes. Drain and immediately rinse with cold water.

In a pan, heat oil over medium heat and sauté onion, garlic and ginger until tender. Add vegetables and sauté 3 to 4 minutes. Stir in cilantro, season with salt and pepper.

In the meantime, soak rice paper in warm water for 30 seconds to 1 minute or until they become soft. Drain and carefully pat dry with a paper towel.

To assemble the spring rolls, place each rice paper on a clean flat surface then place julienned vegetables on one end of the wrap and roll in a cone shape, tucking the wrap in at the bottom.

To serve, place yam onto plates, arrange spring rolls over top, and serve.

Serves 2

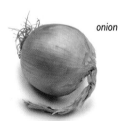

onion

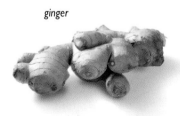

ginger

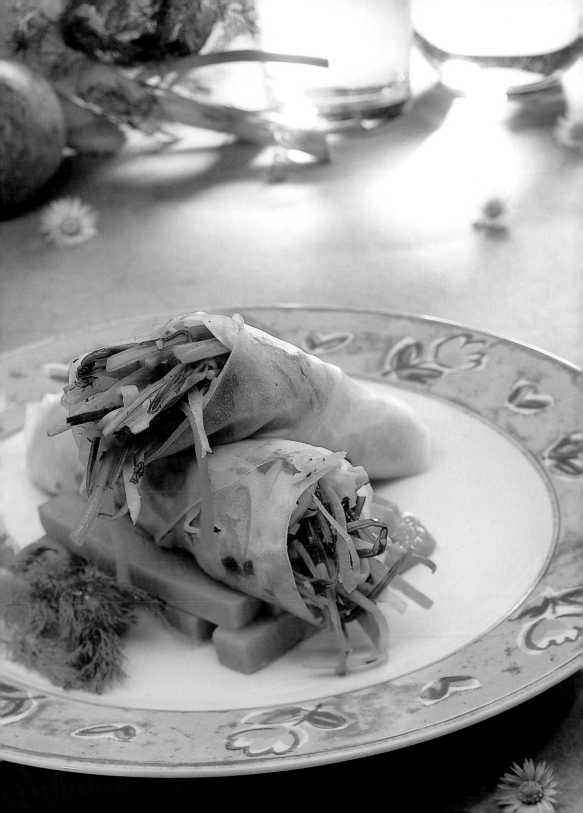

Roasted Vegetables with Wild Rice

Wild rice imparts a distinct flavor and adds a gourmet touch to any meal. This traditional staple of North American natives contains more protein, carbohydrates, minerals and B vitamins than other grains, including wheat, oats or rye.

½ **cup (125 ml) wild rice**

2 ½ **cups (625 ml) water**

½ **cup (125 ml) brown rice**

1 **vegetable bouillon cube**

1 **large zucchini, cut in chunks**

1 **medium squash, cut in chunks**

2-4 **stems baby bok choy**

2 **tbsp coconut oil**

1 **large red onion, quartered**

4-6 **cloves garlic**

In a pot, cook wild rice in water with bouillon for 35 to 40 minutes. Add brown rice and cook for 20 to 25 minutes longer or until all water is absorbed and rice is light and fluffy. Keep warm.

In the meantime, bring a pot of salted water to a boil and blanch zucchini, squash and bok choy for 2 to 3 minutes. Drain and immediately rinse with cold water.

In a pan, heat coconut butter over medium heat and sauté onion, garlic and blanched vegetables for 2 to 3 minutes or until golden brown.

Place vegetables on a platter and serve with the rice.

Serves 2

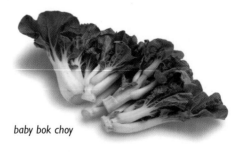

baby bok choy

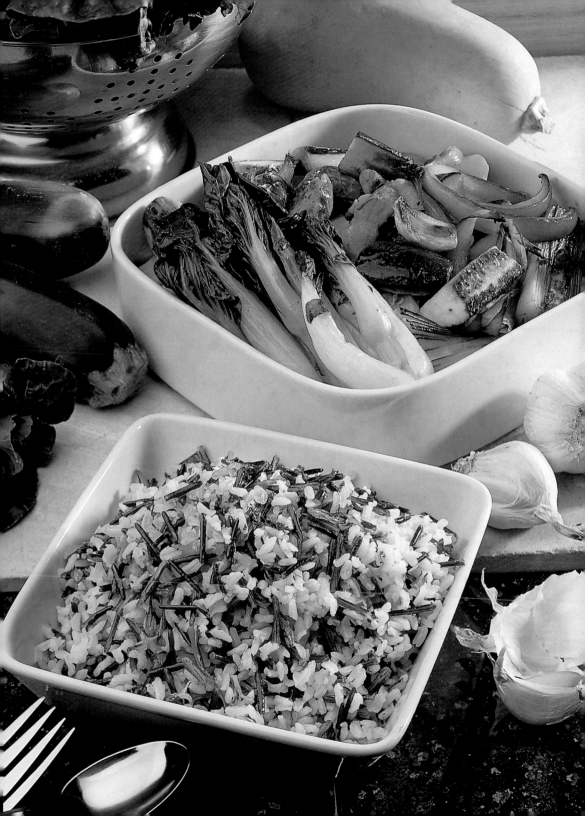

Rice Noodle in Vegetable Broth
with Steamed Root Vegetables

Regularly incorporating root vegetables in the FMS diet will supply you with an abundance of carotenes to ward off damaging free radicals.

I cup (250 ml) **yam, cubed**

I cup (250 ml) **white onion, cubed**

I cup (250 ml) **turnip, cubed**

I cup (250 ml) **celery root, cubed**

I cup (250 ml) **carrots, cubed**

I cup (250 ml) **leek, cut in ½" (I cm) chunks**

I qt (I L) **vegetable stock or water**

2 cups (500 ml) **rice noodles**

Herbamare seasoning, to taste

¼ cup (60 ml) **green onions, chopped, for garnish**

Steam the vegetables in a bamboo or regular steamer for 10 to 12 minutes. Season with salt and pepper.

In the meantime, bring vegetable stock to a boil then pour over rice noodles and let soak for 7 to 10 minutes. Season with salt and pepper, garnish with green onions and serve with the vegetables.

Serves 4

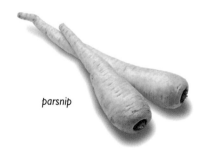

parsnip

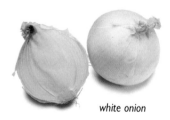

white onion

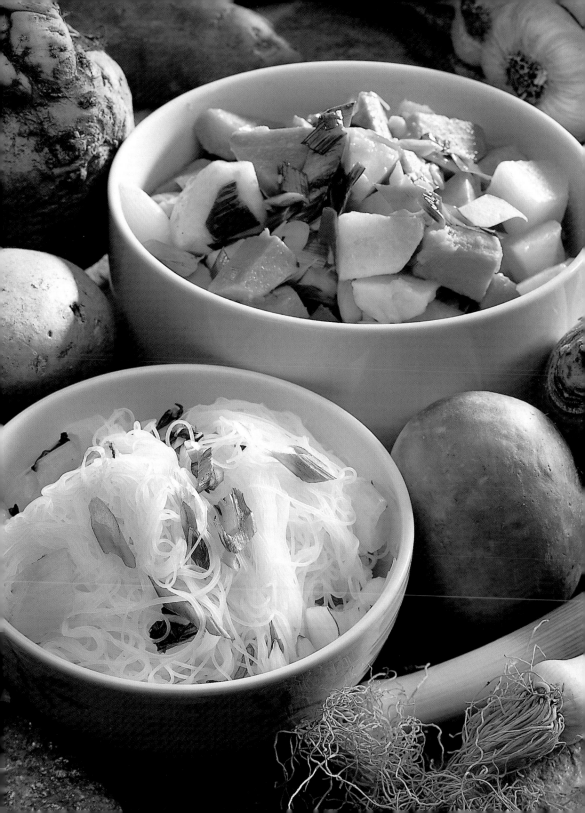

Vegetable Medley

Serve this for a snack or at a party and don't tell your guests you're filling them with free radical-fighting antioxidants. They'll be healthier after enjoying this tasty medley.

1 lb (500 g) asparagus, trimmed

10-12 baby carrots

5 stalks celery, cut 3" (7.5 cm) long

1 cup (250 ml) **cauliflower florets**

1 cup (250 ml) **broccoli florets**

½ cup radish, sliced

2 Belgian endives, leaves separated

You can serve this vegetable medley in various ways. Drizzle with olive oil, toss with seasoning, raw or lightly blanched.

Serves 2

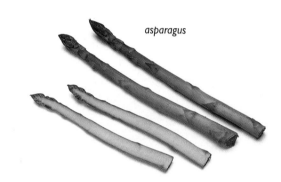

asparagus

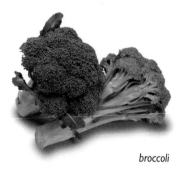

broccoli

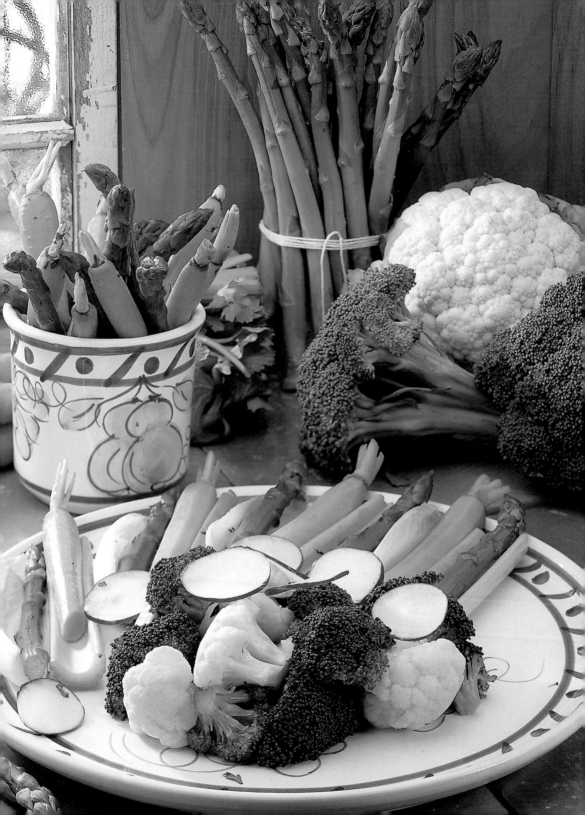

Abraham, G.E., and J.G. Flechas. "Management of fibromyalgia: Rationale for the use of magnesium and malic acid." *Journal of Nutritional Medicine.* 3 (1992): 49-59.

Block, Sydney. "Fibromyalgia and the rheumatisms." *Controversies in Rheumatology.* 19 (1993): 61-78.

Boissevain, M.D., and G.A. McCain. "Toward an integrated understanding of fibromyalgia syndrome. I. Medical and pathophysiological aspects." *Pain.* 45 (1991): 227-238.

Duna, George and William Wilke. "Diagnosis, etiology and therapy of fibromyalgia." *Comprehensive Therapy.* 19:2 (1993): 60-63.

Goldberg, Burton et. al. *Alternative Medicine Guide to Chronic Fatigue, Fibromyalgia & Environmental Illness.* Tiburon: Future Publishing, 1998.

Goldenberg, D.L. "Fibromyalgia and chronic fatigue syndrome: Are they the same?" *Journal of Musculoskeletal Medicine.* 7:19 (1990).

McCain, G.A. et al. "A controlled study of the effects of a supervised cardiovascular fitness training program on manifestations of primary fibromyalgia." *Arthritis Rheum.* 31:1135 (1988).

Moldofsky, H.D. et al. "Musculoskeletal symptoms and non-REM sleep disturbance in patients with 'fibrositis syndrome' and healthy subjects." *Psychosom Med.* 37:341 (1975).

Moldofsky, H.D. "A chronobiologic theory of fibromyalgia." *Journal of Musculoskeletal Pain.* 1:49 (1993).

_____. "Sleep, neuroimmune and neuroendocrine functions in fibromyalgia and chronic fatigue syndrome." *Adv. in Neuroimmunol.* 5 (1995): 39-56.

Romano, T.J. "Magnesium deficiency in fibromyalgia syndrome." *Journal of Nutritional Medicine.* 4:2 (1994): 165-167.

Rona, Zoltan. "Bovine colostrum emerges as immune system modulator." *American Journal of Natural Medicine.* March 1998: 19-23.

Rothschild, Bruce. "Fibromyalgia : An explanation for the aches and pains of the nineties." *Comprehensive Therapy.* 17 (1991): 9-14.

Wolfe, F. et al. "The American College of Rheumatology 1990 criteria for the classification of fibromyalgia: report of the multicenter criteria committee." *Arthritis Rheum.* 33:160 (1990).

Yunus, M.B. et al. "A controlled study of primary fibromyalgia syndrome: Clinical features and association with other functional syndromes." *Journal of Rheumatology* 16(suppl 19):62 (1989).

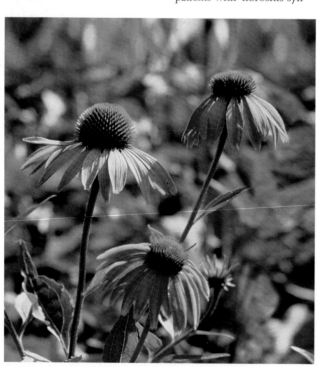

sources

The British Columbia Fibromyalgia Society
P.O. Box 15455
Vancouver, BC
Canada V6B 5B2
Tel: (604) 540-0488
Fax: (604) 520-0481
Email: bcfms@alternatives.com
www.alternatives.com/bcfms

Fibromyalgia Support - Ottawa West (FMS-OW)
Box 26076 - 72 Robertson Road
Nepean, ON
Canada K2H 5Y8
Tel: (613) 831-7129
Fax: (613) 831-6145
Email Coordinator S.C. Alder at:
SCAlder@ncf.ca
www.ncf.ca/fibromyalgia

CFIDS Association of America, Inc.
PO Box 220398
Charlotte, NC 28222-0398
800-442-3437

Fibromyalgia Alliance of America, Inc.
PO Box 21990
Columbus, OH 43221-0990
Tel: (614) 457-4222
Fax: (614) 457-2729
Email: Masaathoff@aol.com

DAMS Inc, Dental Amalgam Mercury Syndrome
Cynthia Saville
856 Sunset Crescent S.E.
Calgary, AB
Canada T2X 3E7
Tel: 1-403-281-5900

Canadians For Mercury Relief
850-36 Toronto Street
Toronto, ON
Canada M5C 2C5
Tel & Fax: (416) 410-6314
www.talkinternational.com

For information on natural health care practitioners across Canada, contact:

Health Action Network Society.
#202 5262 Rumble St.,
Burnaby, BC
Canada V5J 2B6;
Tel: (604) 435-0512
Fax: (604) 435-1561
www.hans.org/
Email: hans@hans.org

Consumer Health Organization of Canada,
1220 Sheppard Ave. E., #412,
Toronto, ON
Canada M2K 2S5;
Tel: (416) 490-0986
Fax: (416) 490-9949
www.consumerhealth.org/home.cfm

Allergy Testing
York Nutritional Laboratory
Murton Way
Osbaldwick, York
YO19 5US,
United Kingdom
Tel: +44 (0) 1904 410410
Fax: +44 (0) 1904 422000
Email: info@allergy.co.uk

Saliva Testing
Some labs in the United States offer saliva testing directly to the public, thereby avoiding the necessity of consulting a doctor. One good lab offering this service to the general public is ZRT Laboratory. You can reach them at:

Tel: (503) 466-2445
Fax: (503) 466-1636
http://www.salivatest.com
ZRT Laboratory
1815 NW 169th Pl. Suite 3090
Beaverton, Oregon 97006

First published in 2000 by
alive books
7436 Fraser Park Drive
Burnaby BC V5J 5B9
(604) 435-1919
1-800-661-0303

© 2000 by alive books

Book Design:
  Liza Novecoski
Artwork:
  Terence Yeung
  Raymond Cheung
Food Styling/Recipe Development:
  Fred Edrissi
Photography:
  Edmond Fong (recipe photos)
  Siegfried Gursche
Photo Editing:
  Sabine Edrissi-Bredenbrock
Editing:
  Sandra Tonn
  Marian MacLean

Canadian Cataloguing in Publication Data

Rona MD, MSc, Zoltan
  Fighting Fibromyalgia

(alive natural health guides, 20
ISSN 1490-6503)
ISBN 1-55312-019-1

Printed in Canada

Revolutionary **Health Books**

alive Natural Health Guides

Each 64-page book focuses on a single subject, is written in easy-to-understand language and is lavishly illustrated with full color photographs.

New titles will be published every month in each of the four series.

Self Help Guides

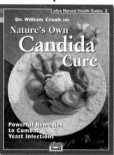

other titles to follow:

- Nature's Own Candida Cure
- Natural Treatment for Chronic Fatigue Syndrome
- Fibromyalgia Be Gone!
- Heart Disease: Save Your Heart Naturally

Healthy Recipes

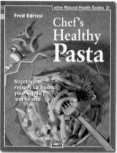

other titles to follow:

- Baking with the Bread Machine
- Baking Bread: Delicious, Quick and Easy
- Healthy Breakfasts
- Desserts
- Smoothies and Other Healthy Drinks

Healing Foods & Herbs

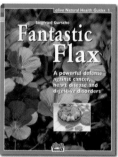

other titles to follow:

- Calendula: The Healthy Skin Helper
- Ginkgo Biloba: The Good Memory Herb
- Rhubarb and the Heart
- Saw Palmetto: The Key to Prostate Health
- St. John's Wort: Sunshine for Your Soul

Lifestyle & Alternative Treatments

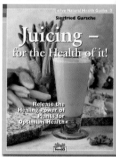

other titles to follow

- Maintain Health with Acupuncture
- The Complete Natural Cosmetics Book
- Kneipp Hydrotherapy at Home
- Magnetic Therapy and Natural Healing
- Sauna: Your Way to Better Health

Vancouver
Canada

Great gifts at an amazingly affordable price **$9.95 Cdn / $8.95 US / £8.95 UK**

alive Natural Health Guides are available in health and nutrition centers and in bookstores. For information or to place orders please dial 1-800-663-6513